When Life Gets Shaky:

Parkinson's
And Life's Trials

By Dale Hansen

Copyright October, 2019

This book is a work of non-fiction.

The reproduction of this book (including copying, scanning, uploading and distribution) without the author's permission, is a theft of the author's property. For permission, please contact the author.

All scripture references and quotations are taken from the New International Study Bible Version (NIV), copyright 1995 by Zondervan Publishing House.

Printed in the USA.

Front and Back cover designs by Mark Beguin.

ISBN # 978-0-578-58378-5

Also by Dale Hansen

"One Day at a Time" (2017)

"Journey Through the Old Testament" (2018)

Includes Dale Hansen

Write Where We Are – WriteOn Joliet Inaugural Anthology (2017)

Write Where We Are – WriteOn Joliet Second Annual Anthology (2018)

Cheetah Stories – a collection of stories, poems and essays based on a silly prompt - a WriteOn Joliet Anthology (2019)

Write Where You Are – WriteOn Joliet Third Annual Anthology (coming 2019)

This book is dedicated to my wife, for her inspiration, encouragement and her ongoing support. She put in many hours of reading, editing and rereading.

Thank you to my readers who encourage me along the way.

Thank you to WriteOn Joliet members for their input, support and growing friendships.

Thank you to my cover illustrator, Mark Beguin.

Thank you to Tom Fry for suggesting using "Shaky" in the book title.

A special thank you to my editors:

Patti Hansen

Heather-Dawn K. Edwards

Allison Dolan

Author Note

This book is based on personal experiences in living with Parkinson's Disease. The Bible verses again, as the verses in my first two Bible devotionals, are verses I have used to challenge, encourage and guide me through living with Parkinson's and through other trials.

This is a life - long process in loving, knowing and obeying God more each day.

I pray my story will give you hope and encouragement through any trials and struggle impacting your many seasons of life.

CONTENTS

Chapter 1	Obedience	Page 1
Chapter 2	Trials	Page 4
Chapter 3	Trust	Page 7
Chapter 4	Mountain	Page 10
Chapter 5	Courageous	Page 13
Chapter 6	Come	Page 16
Chapter 7	Fear	Page 20
Chapter 8	Divine	Page 24
Chapter 9	Prayer	Page 28
Chapter 10	Praise	Page 33
Chapter 11	Glory	Page 36
Epilogue	Intentional	Page 39
Appendix	Parkinson's	Page 41

Chapter 1 Obedience   Genesis 12:1

The LORD had said to Abram, "Go from your country, your people and your father's household to the land I will show you."

Abram (later Abraham) obeyed God by taking his family and leaving his home with no more details on his future. His obedience showed his faith in God.

My wife's best friend was jokingly lying on the ground in front of the moving van in protest of the loading of the van in front of our house. My company offered a transfer to another plant. This would be our first move from Delaware. The decision to move was a hard one but after much prayer, Patti and I decided to accept this offer to move to Rochester. NY. The movers were on their second day of packing the van. We have two daughters. At this time, Bonnie was seven years old and Julie was four years old.

Have you ever made a big decision and then question the decision even when you felt God directed you to your answer? Sometimes change is exciting, but it is hard leaving family and friends behind. This final second day of moving ran into problems with Mother Nature. The morning started with light snow, and the temperatures dropped as the day progressed. Our house was on a slight hill and the truck ramp came up to the house on a slant. The snow caused the ramp to become very slippery and slowed the loading process. The loaders were finally finished filling the truck and pulled out around 6 pm. We left shortly after 6:30 and visited some friends before we left for New York. Up until this age of her life, Julie had given very little indication of any allergy concerns. She also had not been around any cats or dogs. The friends we visited had two large dogs, and Julie's eyes almost immediately swelled shut. We discovered she was allergic to the dogs. The local Emergency Care group gave us medicine and she got better and they sent us on our way around 9 pm. The snow had now turned to sleet and after a quick fast-food pick-up for dinner, we drove about four miles up the road into Pennsylvania and stopped at Ramada Inn for the night. The next day we woke up to a sheet of ice on everything.

This was a shaky beginning! Why were we doing this? Was God with us? Thankfully, He was with us through our obedience! We did leave later in the day and arrived safely in Rochester. It was hard to leave our church in Delaware after eighteen years, and we thought we would never find another similar church we liked. In Rochester, after a few weeks of attending multiple churches, we prayed between two churches and perhaps surprisingly, selected to attend the one that was least like our former church. Our Rochester adventure was well under way.

Moving out of state was a journey with new friends, new church, new neighborhood and new stores. Abram had a similar adventure. As with Abram, God asked him to leave his land, and He obeyed God even though he was given no details. God blessed us as we worked through the details, and we enjoyed our time in Rochester. He proved He was faithful. He was with us, and He could take care of us in a new land with many seasons of joys and challenges ahead of us. Unbeknownst to us, God's future plan for us was to include a challenging new health direction. This would impact our lives forever.

Chapter 2: TRIALS James 1:2

"Consider it pure joy, my brothers and sisters, whenever you face trials of many kinds."

The key word in this verse is "whenever". God does not promise us an easy life as a Christian. What gives us the right to ask for an easy life. We will see trials of many kinds, and He wants us to consider them joyful. The fact is that we grow and learn more in trials and whereas we tend to pull away from Him when all is going well. We consistently need to work on our relationship with God. I have a relationship with my doctor, but I usually only see him when I am sick. My relationship with God should be more than a help number to call. We should seek Him in the midst of all situations. I continually strive to turn a situation over to Him earlier rather than later and trust He will bring me through it. Yet even after decades of walking with the Lord, there are still times when I want to handle things my way. God is not finished with me yet!

After Rochester, God moved us to Joliet, IL, about 45 miles outside of Chicago. We have now lived here for 25 years and have made this our home. Our daughters, sons-in-law and grandkids are here, so we will not be moving anytime soon. My wife and I have an awesome marriage, but we also have had our seasons of struggles. We have worked through infertility issues, breast cancer twice, prostate cancer once, kidney stones and unknown rashes.

I am not trying to suggest this is a heavier or lighter load compared to anyone else's struggles. We all have different challenges come our way as we live our lives. Each of us will also handle them differently. I hope and pray this book will encourage you in all of life's trials, challenges and opportunities.

So how do we find joy in the face of such challenges? Well, the challenge of infertility led to our biggest joys, the adoption of our two wonderful daughters. Of course, we did not greet these health circumstances with open arms. At times we would question God and felt angry. Why us? One lesson we continue to relearn, even today is to trust in Him since He has given us many blessings. In His way He guided us through all of them. The more we waited and trusted God, the more these "opportunities" worked to grow our faith and trust in Him. We do not always understand, but we know He is in control of all areas of our lives. We seek His joy and peace, knowing we will face trials in some seasons of our lives. The above health challenges have great God stories for another time.

The rest of this book will talk about my battle with Parkinson's Disease. Our past experiences with God's faithfulness encouraged us to trust God that this too is part of His plan for us. We do have weak moments, and we work through them. The joy part is, as read, in progress even today. There are times we feel frustrated and discouraged. We have been thoroughly tested already. "God, please leave us alone for a while," we implore. This tested our faith, and as James says, this gave us endurance. I believe God gives us struggles to draw us to Him. You have heard the saying, "God will not give us more than we can handle." I believe this is a myth. I believe He does give us more than we can handle, so we can rely on His strength and not ours. He is always working behind the scenes in our lives even when we are not aware of His presence.

Chapter 3: TRUST Proverbs 3:5,6

"Trust in the LORD with all your heart
and lean not on your own understanding;
in all your ways submit to him,
and he will make your paths straight".

God is asking for complete trust with all our hearts. During struggles in my life, I try to be intentional to trust in Him completely and try not to ask for specific answers or attempt to understand how He will answer or work. I know He loves me and wants to be the leader of my life. He wants us to submit to him, allow Him to work His purpose in our lives and not to stray off His path and His direction. We sometimes want to go our way and then ask Him to bless our way. We must first pray to find His way and purpose, so He can and will help us with His way. I believe prayer may change us and not just change the circumstances.

The diagnosis of Parkinson's disease was a whole new challenge for me. Many of the health issues Patti and I have already worked through have better known names somewhat familiar to us.

Parkinson's, however was different. There are so many variations of Parkinson's with each person presenting different symptoms. The most common symptoms include shaking/ movement issues, balance/ strength issues and mental/ memory issues. Those living with Parkinson's may deal with one set or a combination of issues. For example, some friends have mental issues with no shaking, while some have mental and strength issues with no shaking. Although this disease can be somewhat managed, researchers are still looking for a cure and they are far from understanding it. All I knew at first was parts of my body were shaking off and on uncontrollably, and I did not know why it was happening.

I was diagnosed in 2004 with tremors and began to learn about uncontrolled body movements. Initially I just lived with the shaking since my symptoms were not interfering with my daily activities and living. One year later, as my shaking became worse, my diagnosis was changed to Parkinson's disease. As we prayed and focused on trusting God, He began to answer in His way. We knew He would guide us through this. Although God can cure all diseases, we felt that may not be part of His plan for us at this time.

As we consider God's plan, a few summers ago, Patti and I took a road trip from Joliet, IL back to the east coast to visit family, cousins and friends. We had a general schedule and made no hotel reservations ahead of time. Well, some nights we had trouble finding hotels and wished we had a better plan. If we do a road trip again, we will have a plan. Certainly, at the beginning, we had no initial plan for our Parkinson's trip. For this medical trip, we had no idea what was ahead, what questions to ask or what impact this would have on our future.

The hard part of praying during these times was the many unknowns, with very few specifics. However, Patti and I look back at our 30-plus year walk with God and know we can trust Him and give our worries to Him. I found that through Parkinson's, God continues to strengthen and grow my trust and faith in Him. In many situations, God may not always resolve the situation right away, but we found His peace and support every day. We watched for His timing and learned more of His plan as the weeks and months unfolded.

Chapter 4: MOUNTAIN   Matthew 17:20

"He replied, "Because you have so little faith. Truly I tell you, if you have faith as small as a mustard seed, you can say to this mountain, 'Move from here to there,' and it will move. Nothing will be impossible for you."

Our faith is often tested to ensure our complete trust in God. He does not always answer our prayers the way we want. Part of our relationship with Him is knowing this and following Him more each day. Our prayers seeking our desires should then begin to match closer to what He desires for our lives. He may answer in ways we do not expect, and He may not always move the mountain we may perceive in our lives. We must see this as an opportunity to grow our trust and faith in God. Patti and I experienced some anxiety, and I did some reading about Parkinson's. Based on our prayers, the reading and what we believed God's plan was for us, we decided not to start with any medicines at that time. After my diagnosis was changed to Parkinson's in 2005, I tried not to show my shaking in public. Eventually,

I realized God wanted me to share my condition. I found everyone already noticed something was up with me. If you are in a similar challenge or struggle, I encourage you to share with others to get valuable encouragement and prayer support, as those around you already see something is going on. Through my sharing I was able to get in touch with others who have the disease to learn more about it. One patient had the Deep Brain Stimulation (DBS) surgery which could be one potential possibility for my shaking. You could not even tell that he had Parkinson's. I will explain later DBS in chapter six. My wife and I were wondering what our future would look like. As this was hard to admit we believed God had a unique plan for us.

For the first 5 years, with God's help, I managed without medicines. However, my motor symptoms continued to worsen until I could not keep my hands very steady and my left leg shook a lot. My energy level continued to drop due to my shaking as did my weight. All this was very frustrating and discouraging. At this point, it became clear God wanted us to begin to start trying medicines. Some worked, some stopped working and some did not help at all. Some of them actually gave me symptoms of the disease. I continued as God moved me through the doctor visits and the medicine monitoring. As mentioned earlier, doctors still do not understand Parkinson's disease. My mountain (Parkinson's) may remain, but He gave me the wisdom, strength and support from others to deal with the mountain. I was motivated to spend more time to know God better as this disease progressed.

Sometimes God will move the mountain and heal you. The God today is the same God performing miracles for His people Israel and showing His power in the Old Testament. We came to realize God's plan for us was to deal with the mountain. We may not understand why some are cured of Parkinson's or any health issues and some are not cured. We must always remember that nothing is impossible with God.

Chapter 5:   COURAGEOUS   Joshua 1:9

"Have I not commanded you? Be strong and courageous. Do not be afraid; do not be discouraged, for the LORD your God will be with you wherever you go."

Synonyms for courageous include brave, bold, adventurous and fearless. Antonyms to courageous include fearful and shaky. In Joshua 1, God is preparing Joshua and his people to go into the unknown Promised Land and the Lord will be with them. Just like Abraham, Joshua was not given any details for this move. All Joshua knew was there would be lots of milk and honey. Unfortunately, from the scouts first report of the land, there were giants in the land and the people's first reaction was negative. "We will never defeat them", they moaned. In our situation, Parkinson's sounded overwhelming like the report of giants. This was all new territory. We prayed as we worked through different medicines and potential surgery decisions as we lived through each day. This was an adventure and one that we did not sign up for, and we did stumble at times in the process. Our emotions ranged from scared of where this path was leading, to knowing this was not a simple fix and to joy knowing we were making progress on His path. God was still involved, of course. He was not surprised with what unfolded. He was with us and challenged us to follow Him and be brave and bold.

Our prayer life grew and yet there were still some weak moments during this time. We prayed and the situation actually became worse before it improved as our faith was tested. Sometimes we had to refocus our trust in Him. We sought Him with hope and intentionally spent more time in His Word for encouragement, rather than just praying, "woe is me".

We resolved to be courageous, believing we could work through this disease with God. At times, we looked for quicker progress, but as always, we had to wait for His timing. Sometimes as we commit to follow God, He challenges us to wait and make sure we really trust Him. We must be reminded that our first priority is still our relationship with Him. All of our prayers are building a relationship and not just a request line. We often do well when life is good, but we struggle when our lives get tough. These hard times draw us closer to Him. In our case, we could look back and be reassured as we had Him help us through prior struggles. We still do not understand the why and what of Parkinson's. Just like Joshua had to challenge the people to be brave and bold following God into the Promised Land, Patti and I prayed to be brave as He moved us forward into a future we did not know. Israel was promised the land, but it was not promised to be easy. God wanted them to conquer the people already in the land. God wants us out of our comfort zone. Then our reliance will be on His divine power and not ourselves. Joshua used the word "courageous" in four verses in chapter 1 of Joshua. The emphasis is on being strong, staying fearless and not getting discouraged. God is with us wherever we go. We may not always feel His presence, but He is still there. He was with Abraham and Joshua. God was also with Patti and I as we worked through this Parkinson's journey. One of my favorite short prayers, is "Lord, help me to be more aware of your presence each day!"

Chapter 6:   COME   Matthew 11:28

"Come to me, all you who are weary and burdened, and I will give you rest".

Matthew starts this verse with. "Come to me". Jesus wants all who are weary with life to come to Him, and He will provide rest. Coming to Christ is the top priority we should have in our lives. Although He does listen to our daily requests and He does want our relationship to be more important to Him and for us. He first loves us and desires us to know Him and to talk to Him more in prayer. When I am having a hard day or hard season, I intentionally spend more quiet time with Him to refocus on Him only. I do not ask for anything, I praise Him or pray for others. This is very hard to do. However, I lay my issues before Him, and I can then allow Him to give me rest. At this point, we decided to continue with different medicines. For the next two years I worked with my doctor on the Parkinson's medicines. My shaking was still noticeable. My energy level continued to be low due to the energy used when shaking, and I lost a great deal of weight. Resting in God helped restore me. After limited progress with the different medicines, God led me to get a second opinion. I switched doctors and began trying other medicines and varying the dosages. I saw some improvements over the next four years. After a while some of the medicines would stop working. Some of the dosages were crazy. Smaller amounts but more dosages throughout the day. They were difficult to keep up with, and I always missed some each day. Additionally, some of the side effects of the medicines aggravated the Parkinson's symptoms. The official term is dyskinesia where higher dosages of certain Parkinson's medicines can increase movements or shaking. Our next option was to consider surgery. One of the advantages of surgery is a consistent stimulation 24 hours per day versus irregular pill taking. The doctor thought in my case I should look into surgery since my symptoms were all exclusively shaking. I showed no signs of strength, balance or mental issues. DBS (Deep Brain Stimulation) surgery helps most with the shaking, and we were told this was typically very effective. This surgery is in two parts. Part one was four and a half hours of brain surgery. Part two, a few days later, was a one-hour surgery of implanting a power pack in my chest.

We had been hoping and trusting God with the medicines. My personal time with Him encouraged me. God was moving us into a different season of our lives (retirement). We continued to pray about the next few years. DBS surgery sounded very scary. I was sent to the Movement Disorder Department at Rush Hospital in Chicago to be evaluated. We continued to be directed to a new God adventure, and Patti and I prayed we would be courageous looking toward Rush Hospital and the great unknown.

We visited Rush hospital almost every other month and communicated with them almost every month as we monitored how the medicines were working or not working. We saw very little progress over almost one year, and God began to guide us to consider the DBS (Deep Brain Stimulation)

We laid this before God to take this burden and came to Him for peace about the surgery decision. One of the ways we always have cleared our heads when life challenges overwhelm us to get away into nature. One of our favorite spots is Starved Rock Park near Utica, IL. This park has many trails, canyons and overlooks and is only about an hour away. A one-day trip typically includes a hike in the morning, another in the afternoon with a nice lunch at the Lodge between our hikes. Sometimes we bring books to read. Although we are confident God is still with us, this time away helps us to refocus and we want to keep our relationship with God as a priority. Now we needed to make a potential life changing decision on the surgeries, and I was overwhelmed with fear.

Chapter 7: FEAR   Psalm 34:4

"I sought the Lord, and he answered me;
  he delivered me from all my fears."

As anxiety and outright fear almost overwhelmed me, Patti and I continued to give our questions about this to the Lord. I did not want to continue to be shaky! How do you seek whatever He wants for our lives when you do not see the purpose or reason for what He may have us go through? We confirmed by trusting that God was in control and would deliver us from our fears. We were dependent on God and thankful for His guidance in the past.

As the medicine's effectiveness continued to drop, my overall energy level also continued to drop. I was very slow at getting dressed or undressed, tying my shoes, and taking a shower. It was like driving at 30 MPH and everyone around me was driving at 70 MPH. I started to take more naps. At this point, I could not sit for very long and my legs would start to shake. I struggled at times sitting for a Bible study or through a church service. Yet, through this, we prayed and God directed us to go forward with the DBS surgeries. This final major decision was confirmed with prayer. We scheduled the two surgeries about four days apart in September, 2017. Rush hospital did a very good job with the initial information, the surgery, the recovery and follow ups after I went home. Through this process, Patti influenced change in one of the steps in the surgery prep process at the hospital. In preparation for the surgery, they drilled a square head brace (halo) into my head with screws. As a result, my head was bleeding (although it did not hurt). However, it was horrible to see and Patti asked them to clean the blood which they finally did after she kept asking. When the hospital asked for feedback, Patti told them about this situation. She suggested family members should be warned and told what was coming. Then they can decide whether or not they want to remain in the room. And with or without family present, the person's head should be cleaned. The hospital now follows this procedure.

I belong to a writer's group, WriteOn Joliet which has an open mic night two times a year, and one recent topic was Fear. I read the following story titled "Don't Take a Nap":

"I started to doze and I heard one of the doctor's say no time for napping. I was in surgery for my Parkinson's. I heard the steady hum of the computer and could barely see the screen showing my brain waves. Good. At least I had brain waves. Earlier, they locked a halo on my head. With surgery underway my halo felt a little tight but at least my head was clean of any blood. My head could not move at all, as they checked the different wire hook ups to my brain. After an hour, I was afraid I could not make it to the end of this surgery. As I again tried to doze, a doctor repeated don't take a nap. We need you to stay awake. Raise your right leg. They wanted to make sure my brain didn't tell my left arm to go up. Then some good news. We are about half done. Great. Good news? Easy for them to say. Only another 2 ¼ more hours.

We prayed about this surgery and felt God wanted me to take care of my Parkinson's. I am in overall good health. I am a runner and have a high tolerance of pain. Yet, I still needed to trust in Him to handle this surgery. I went over Bible verses in my head as He led me fearlessly through the final hours. Okay, Dale, we are almost done. I do not want to catch you napping. Your brain waves will tell us if you doze off. Busted – no napping. A computer is watching me. Now, raise your right hand. Good. My right hand went up. Almost done. Then I hear those wonderful words: We are done and the surgery went very well. Now recovery, surgery the following week for the power pack (Definitely asleep for that one!), programming, multiple visits and now 97% percent free of Parkinson's symptoms. Love modern technology and thank God for this process. Think I will take a nap".

Dale Hansen   10/07/2017

I take very few naps now and my energy level continues to remain at a good level with no slowness and little shaking. God is great, mighty and powerful.

Chapter 8: DIVINE 2 Peter 1:3

"His divine power has given us everything we need for a godly life through our knowledge of him who called us by his own glory and goodness."

2 Peter tells us we have access to God's divine power for living a godly life through knowing and praising Him. What a source of power at our disposal as He calls us through His glory and goodness. If we follow Him, He will provide us with all we need each day and in each season of life.

As mentioned earlier, my deep brain stimulation was a two-part surgery. Part one was four and a half hours involving connecting wires to both sides of my brain, and I needed to stay awake during this time. Four electrodes were attached and run from my brain to a power pack in my left chest area. These would run a steady electrical signal to my brain 24/7 at an adjustable dose. The adjustments would control the right and left sides of my brain.

Part two was placing the battery power pack (similar to a heart monitor) in my chest and connecting the electrodes from my brain. This was a one-hour surgery, and I was put to sleep. I was very happy to sleep during that surgery. The power pack would stimulate my brain with a steady dose and would be adjustable.

One of the major disadvantages of the medicines I had been taking was sporadic dosing which does not help as much as a lower but steady dosage. The power pack dosage is able to continue to be adjusted and regulated, and doctors believe this steady dosage can reduce the symptoms very dramatically over time.

The next step after the surgery was visiting the office at Rush Hospital about a month later to turn the power pack on and start making adjustments to reach the best results. With all the combinations and two sides to regulate, the doctors said this would take about six months. After the pack was initially turned on, my energy came back instantly. Within two weeks, I was back to running a few days a week. Over the next few months, adjustments continued to be made. I was even given some ability to make adjustments myself but with limitations.

Given the success of the surgery, I was invited to participate in some government funded research.

Rush Hospital referred me to Northwestern Hospital for this research. So, in June, 2018, I went to Northwestern in Chicago for some baseline tests. Testing included eye/ hand movement, overall strength, memory, gait and arm/ leg strength. This government grant paid for a five-day stay in Chicago for Patti and me. We were excited to help in this research. I visited the hospital for about four hours each day for the testing. The rest of the day was free time, and we spent some time walking around the city and the lake front and saw a play. Follow up to this research project will happen around the Fall of 2021, and they will look for any changes versus the original base tests. I am doing this to help bring hope to future Parkinson's patients.

This was literally brain surgery. We prayed and talked to two former patients for more insight about both surgeries before we made a decision to do this. We trusted we would make the right decision. Through our relationship with God, He has given us access to His divine power. That is all we need to live a Godly life through our knowledge of Him. This is the same power used to part the Red Sea, save Daniel in the lion's den, raise Lazarus from the dead, and guide my wife and me in dealing with my Parkinson's. His divine nature can keep us safe from the evil desires of this world on a daily basis and in all moments. His power can help us with whatever plans He has for us. For Patti and me, this included Parkinson's and the two surgeries. We do not always understand or make the right decisions. But through our years together, we have seen God work in our lives, and we always hope and pray our faith is growing.

Chapter 9: PRAYER

"Let us acknowledge the LORD; let us press on to acknowledge him. As surely as the sun rises, he will appear; he will come to us like the winter rains, like the spring rains that water the earth." Hosea 6:3

"Devote yourselves to prayer, being watchful and thankful." Colossians 4:2

"Keep this Book of the Law always on your lips; meditate on it day and night, so that you may be careful to do everything written in it. Then you will be prosperous and successful." Joshua 1:8

I would like to take this chapter off to detour from my story, and focus on my prayer life. Prayer has played a vital role in keeping me tuned into God, seeking his guidance and growing my faith. As God has guided me through many different seasons, joys and trials in my life, my time in prayer has evolved. It is very different from years ago. I do praise Him more to begin with, and I am very thankful for what He has done in the past and continues to do in my life today. My prayer life has always been a priority, except now I believe I focus more on strengthening my relationship with God instead of just coming to Him with my requests or only when I need His help. I keep on being reminded I must go to Him first rather than ask for His help after I have messed things up doing things my way. Sometimes, I fail to pray and involve Him before making a decision or taking action. The lesson that I must follow His lead and involve Him from the beginning has needed to be repeated.

The best thing I did to enhance my prayer life was to stop reading books about prayer and how to pray, and just started praying. There is no one-size-fits all approach to prayer. I learned to trust that God would lead me in this area as well. I started a prayer list with dates and answers, almost like a journal. That is a praise in itself since I am normally not a "journaler." Sometimes I pray regularly (daily) and, other times I pray more often throughout the day. I am still a work in progress, and my goal is to have a consistent daily prayer life and walk with God.

The three verses above, reference three key themes for prayer:

1) Seeking to know Him,
2) A devoted prayer life
3) Staying in His Word.

As Hosea says we must seek to know Him more, and He will come to us. He will come as sure as the morning sun and spring rains will appear. This is His promise as we press to get to know Him better. We must get to know Him by spending some time with Him.

A key way to spend time with Him is prayer. We must be fully devoted to our relationship with God and with our prayer time with Him. I am not talking of a quick "here are my requests" prayer. We need to strive for a more meaningful and disciplined conversational prayer time. In addition, we should leave time to listen in silence for His response. This has been a slow process as I continue to grow in faith. I am seeing some improvements as I continue to seek more meaningful and sincere times in prayer. Prayer takes discipline, hard work and motivation and must be intentional. These factors work together. My prayer time draws me closer to God and, knowing God better helps my prayer time. Of course, spending time in His Word can enhance our prayer time. We can start by selecting from the many prayers found in the book of Psalms. They cover many topics including praise, thanks, seeking forgiveness and guidance. Using Biblical prayers can encourage and support you in current and future opportunities. Time in His Word can help you build a solid foundation in growing your relationship with God. Personally, I have built a pack of about 110 verses. These are some key verses that have helped me through the years. Sometimes my time with the Lord is reading and praying through these verses. I still add verses as God reveals them to me. All of this is an ongoing process as I move through the many seasons and challenges of my life.

We should also include some close friends for their prayer support, and in turn we can also pray for them. My current prayer list includes seven people that have started new jobs recently and seven more looking for new jobs. My closest friend is my wife, Patti. We started praying together consistently by setting an alarm for 8 pm each night to remind us. Now we can remind each other and do not use an alarm. We should always be on the lookout for ways to grow our prayer lives and intentionally spending more time with Him. After we spend time with Him in prayer or in His Word, we can allow God to respond to us – as sure as tomorrow's morning sun.

Chapter 10:   PRAISE   Job 38:11

"When I said, 'This far you may come and no farther; here is where your proud waves halt'?"

Overall, for Patti and I, our prayer time has grown during these years with our different health issues. We want to give God all the praise. The first part of our prayer times begin with praise and thanks to our God. He is God. He has stayed with us in the past to help us through various trials and is present in our lives today, and we are confident in His presence and guidance in our future. This has been a long process, but we are reminded God is all powerful, all knowing and all loving. Job 38 reminds us He is in control. God responds to Job questioning who is in control. This is a great chapter to read and meditate on, with my favorite verse in this chapter being verse 11. This includes commanding where each wave breaks on the shore. This verse inspired me to write the following poem, which talks about the waves in all our seasons of life. God has control of the waves, the seas and the rivers, along with any crisis in any season of our lives. The title is "Waves of Life":

Waves always on the move

White caps with no patterns

Power currents sweep you away

Quiet ripples put you to sleep.

Deep is never for the weak

Careful as it overwhelms

Mighty waves must beware

Gentle waves for the calm.

God knows our daily living

He'll keep us above the waves

Will help us through the waves

And lead us to calm waters.

God does control the waves

And commands every one

He knows where they'll stop

No further they will go.

Trust in Him and sense His soothe

Waves of life are on the move

Dale Hansen   03/22/2019

God has been and is still with us when we are overcome by waves. Looking back, we can see how God performed a miracle for us thanks to our friends' prayer support, to the people at Rush Hospital and to modern research and technology.

Chapter 11: GLORY Revelation 4:11

"You are worthy, our Lord and God, to receive glory and honor and power, for you created all things, and by your will they were created and have their being." Revelation 4:11

God has been with Patti and me and is still with us in this adventure. Even when we were concerned, afraid and very unsure, He did not change or leave us. At times, it was hard to keep pressing through, but God helped us grow our trust and faith in Him. We give Him all the glory and praise. When you drive with Jesus in your "car of life", you need to keep reading His Word and pray. We must keep the car moving. A car parked on the side of the road goes nowhere and accomplishes nothing. When the car is moving, we may swerve to the right or left at times, but He can direct us back to the lane we need to be in. We continue to move ahead while waiting for His answers, spending time in His Word and time in prayer.

Since the surgery, we have visited Rush Hospital monthly with ongoing adjustments to the power pack. As of May 1, 2019, a full twenty months after the surgery, only my head was shaking a little. I had not needed to make adjustments the last couple months. From time to time, I made small adjustments on my left side to reduce the head shaking and ensure all other areas were still. I also visit Rush periodically to make additional adjustments. My energy level reached 110%, I gained some weight and sleep well except for some periodic hallucinations. My mental functions and strength remain good. I am thankful that for now I have reached a point where I am only dealing with some slight head shaking. We give Him all the praise and glory as we continue to move forward. With God as the leader of our lives and allowing Him to work through us, we have immeasurably accomplished more than we could have ever dreamed or imagined.

He is the Creator and knows and controls all things. He continues to lead us daily through this new territory. This disease affects each person in different ways and in different severities. This makes it difficult to understand, educate people about Parkinson's and communicate new information. There are experts in the field, including Parkinson's and Movement Disorder groups, which share recent research findings. For example, recent studies have suggested constipation may be an early sign of this disease. A doctor with limited knowledge may not know to connect the two. Many studies have found exercise may help reduce the symptoms, at least short term, and potentially longer. These exercises include running, bike riding, karate and boxing.

We continue to hope for more technological advancement to learn more on how to reduce the symptoms, have better understanding, find a cure and completely eliminate Parkinson's for future generations.

Epilogue: INTENTIONAL

My journey continues today and Patti and I continue to work on our relationship and time with God. I can sit for longer periods of time with no legs shaking, and leading a men's Bible study. Since my operation, I have written and published two devotionals as well as working on this book. I also have been posting a 'Video Verse of the week" every Tuesday on Facebook. I trained and ran two 5-K races in the spring. Patti and I recently drove a 2100 mile and eight state road trip. All hotels were planned and booked ahead of time, along with confirming dates and a full itinerary of our trip. This made a big difference in our enjoyment of the trip, compared to our earlier poorly planned trip.

Every day is a new day and a new adventure in our walk with God. We never know and may not understand what God has in store for us for the rest of our lives – whether it is 20 or 30 years. We do know He loves us, desires a relationship with us, and will never leave us or forsake us. Over the past decades, and the more recent years dealing with Parkinson's Disease, God has a plan for us. We continue to hold on to our relationship with Him as we obey Him and seek His guidance.

We did strive to adjust our lives through many situations including two out of state moves, infertility, breast cancer twice, kidney stones and most recently, prostate cancer.

My favorite word is "intentional". I want to be intentional in my actions. For example, I work at being intentional with making phone calls for encouragement, praying for someone I promised I would pray for, spending time with God and growing my faith.

I pray all of us make the right big and small choices we are confronted with each day, knowing God is with us even if we are not sure.

Will we choose His way or our way?

Appendix: PARKINSON'S DISEASE

WHAT IS PD?

- Starts with the death of cells in a certain part of the brain.
- Dopamine is in these cells and is now at a lower level in the brain.
- Dopamine is a neurotransmitter.
- Dopamine is responsible for relaying messages which plan and control body movement.
- A dopamine deficiency means less control of body movements.

FACTS

- The cause of this disease is still unknown.
- It appears to happen randomly, with few traces to heredity.
- There is no cure.
- Each person can have different motor symptoms which may include tremors, slow movement, balance, swallowing issues and smaller handwriting.
- Many people can have non-movement symptoms including mood disorders, cognitive issues, fatigue, sleep disorders and hallucinations.
- There are medications, and in some cases, surgery, which may delay the development of Parkinson's.
- Life adjustments, including medications and exercise can help a patient to lead a good quality life style.

Thank you for reading this story. Can you please go and review this book on Amazon. This would be a big help. Thank you in advance.

I would love any feedback on this story.

My e-mail is:

Dale1873@gmail.com

For more information about my books and myself, please visit my website:

www.groundedandgrowingweekly.com

Friend me on Facebook to see my "VIDEO VERSE of the week" every Tuesday.

LIST OF VERSES/ NOTES:

Made in the USA
Lexington, KY
09 November 2019